M000094093

This guided recovery workbook evolved from 17+ years as a Medical Intuitive, with special focus on Chronic Lyme. Healing Lyme disease involves spiritual initiation and a soul recovery process. I designed this workbook to help you complete your initiation - to nurture soul, creativity, and the most authentic you.

This workbook supports different levels of the healing process, but is not intended to replace medical or other therapeutic advice. By reading and responding to these questions, you accept responsibility for your own journey, and the author disclaims all liability. Your answers are yours and yours alone. All questions are copyrighted to Laura Bruno, 2018. All rights reserved.

1. What skills, talents, attitudes, personality traits, and/or gifts do you already have, and which new ones are you developing? What's "right" with you? Take inventory and offer thanks.

2. What coincidences, signs or synchronicities have you noticed lately? Have you had any recurring "random" thoughts, conversations or dreams? What small details suggest a larger theme?

3. In one word, how do you feel about your illness? In one word, what's the feeling about your illness behind that feeling? Now, what's the feeling behind both of those feelings? Explore that third feeling about your illness. Does it surprise you? Why or why not? How does this third feeling shed light on your healing journey?

4. What does your intuition tell you that you need for your recovery? How can you address these needs? What small step(s) can you take towards following your intuition today? This week? This month?

5. Do you want to ask the usual people for help, or would you feel better with different avenues of support? Why do you feel this way?

6. What small action would feel like a celebration just for you, just for now? Will you give yourself permission to take this small action? Why or why not? If not, then which small, celebratory action will you allow yourself to take? Do it.

7a. In what ways do you allow yourself to shine regardless of weather, news, or your surroundings? How do you feel when you allow yourself to shine?

7b. In what ways do you dim yourself to blend in with other people or expectations? List three "stealth" ways to shine. Which symbolic actions feel bright inside yourself even if no one notices?

8a. If you had a calling or life path, what would it be? In what ways have you already lived this path, and in what ways do you long to deepen your experience?

8b. Even if you don't know your life path, make a list of things that attract or intrigue you. Soul whispers in quiet longings and simple delight. Listen.

9a. What fundamental beliefs structure your reality and options? In which ways do these beliefs support or impede your recovery?

9b. Playing Devil's Advocate, can you find any wiggle room, tweaks or experimental "what if's" to undermine beliefs that undermine your health?

10. Would you rather be right or be well? Why? What does your answer tell you about your recovery process? How can you use this information to improve your healing strategy?

11a. What are the differences between "attachment," "detachment" and "non-attachment"? Which state feels stressful? Which state feels isolated? Which state allows for joyful surprises?

11b. What attitudes, habits and actions would support more freedom, flexibility and joyful surprises in your life?

12a. What's the difference between "acceptance" and "settling"? How do they feel in your mind, body, and heart?

12b. When you accept or decisively reject something, what does that decision free you to do?

13a. Imagine Lyme as a spiritual initiation: what kind of position or path might you be initiated into?

13b. Which Guides or Helpers have you encountered? What Guardians of the Treasure have you met? What kind of treasure requires strong guardians?

13c. What if you were "chosen" instead of "punished" by Lyme disease? How would this information change your approach to healing?

14a. Are you more critical of yourself or others? Why? Do you feel judged? Do you judge people for judging you? Do you judge yourself for judging others?

14b. How does your body feel when you judge yourself or others?

15. What habits, affirmations or strategies would help you to feel less reactive? Explore different types of reactivity, i.e. physical/autoimmune reactions, emotional reactivity, confusion, etc.

16a. What does "Respect, Not Control" mean to you? How do these concepts affect your relationships?

16b. Do you aim for respect, control, or a combination? Why?

16c. How do your attitudes towards respect and control affect your relationship with yourself? Your symptoms?

17a. Do you trust your doctors and caregivers? Why or why not?

17b. What would help you to feel more empowered on your healing journey?

18a. If tomorrow brought a complete, spontaneous healing, what would you do? How would you feel?

18b. What would "prove" to you that you had healed?

18c. What small or symbolic activity can you do each day that reminds you of that "proof" of your own healing?

19a. If tomorrow brought a complete, spontaneous healing, what decisions would you need to make that don't seem like possible choices right now?

19b. What kind of support would you need in order to make the most empowering decisions? Affirm that you accept and receive the support you need for the Highest Good of All, including you.

20a. Who or what haunts you? Why and how does the haunting occur?

20b. What would give you (or them) closure (i.e. a letter, conversation, ceremony, visit, symbolic action)? Brainstorm ways you can lay these ghosts to rest.

21a. What should's and must's rule your life? Do these expectations provide welcome structure, or do they feel restrictive?

.

21b. What do your should's and must's reveal about your values?

22a. Which relationships demand more of you than you receive in return? Is this a temporary, new development, or a long term pattern?

22b. How do imbalanced relationships affect your symptoms, energy, and emotions? What's in it for you?

22c. What relationship boundaries or support do you need for your healing?

23a. What animal dreams, coincidences, and encounters have you experienced?

23b. On a symbolic level, what might they be trying to tell you?

24a. If you were an animal, what would you be and why?

24b. What qualities of your chosen animal do you possess, and which ones would you love to have at your disposal? How would those additional qualities help you heal and enjoy your life?

25a. Do you ever feel guilty about taking time to care for yourself? Why or why not?

25b. What small steps or personal mantras would help you to feel more balanced and supported?

26a. How do you experience time? Does it cycle, spiral, vary pace, or always proceed in the same direction at the same rate?

26b. What's the difference between "time" and "timing"?

27a. In which areas of life do you experience reactivity?

27b. What's the difference between reacting, responding, and embracing? Which feels better in your body?

28a. What thoughts, emotions, foods, attitudes and/or situations trigger increased symptoms? What themes and patterns do you notice in this list?

28b. Are these new in your life, or amplified old themes and patterns? Under what circumstances did they first begin?

28c. If symptoms were guiding you to improve your life, towards which directions and decisions do improved symptoms point?

29a. List some experiences that initially seemed bad but turned out to be blessings in disguise.

29b. What potential blessings can you find in your current challenges? What would be a surprisingly lovely outcome?

30a. List five reasons you feel grateful for your healing journey. What surprises you about this list, and why?

30b. How do you feel when you express gratitude?

31a. To what other options might your closed doors be pointing you? Can you find a window, a portal or an unexplored doorway?

31b. What door do you hope appears? How would crossing that threshold feel?

32a. In what ways do you embody a need for generational healing?

32b. With names, photos, or family tree, ponder and describe how your lineage runs through your life. How do your life challenges represent larger patterns in need of healing?

32c. How does this awareness of generational patterns shift your attitude and healing strategy?

33a. What event in the past do you wish you had not witnessed? What dynamics of this event continue to play out in your life?

33b. Do you need to forgive yourself or anyone else related to this event or these dynamics? Before you go to sleep tonight, ask your subconscious to reclaim any pieces of your soul lost in this event.

34a. What superpower do you wish you had? What unusual or freakish "gifts" do you already have?

34b. In which ways do you sometimes dim your light in order to appear more "normal" than you are? What do you think would happen if you allowed yourself to shine?

35a. What real life heroes inspire you and why?

35b. What qualities do you share with these heroes? Which qualities do you intend to develop?

36a. What are your favorite comeback stories or films? When have you triumphed when you thought you might fail?

36b. What thoughts and habits comfort you and strengthen your resolve?

37a. Have you ever been sexually harassed or sexually abused? If so, do you feel you've healed from this? What other kinds of abuse or boundary violations have you experienced?

37b. Do you feel supported to move through these issues? If not, what kind of support would help you to heal on all levels?

37c. What would you need in order to forgive the abuser and yourself?

38a. Name something for which you feel guilty or ashamed. At that time and that level of awareness, what other options did you have? Why did you choose as you did?

.

38b. What pieces of you remain linked to guilt or shame? Before you go to sleep tonight, intend and ask your subconscious to reclaim any pieces of your soul stuck in this experience.

39a. Which "helpful people" in your life actually make you feel worse? Which relationship dynamics negatively impact your health or peace of mind? Be honest.

39b. Brush each arm from shoulder down past your fingertips, alternating arms, three times each. Flick your fingers three times like you just washed your hands, and there's no towel. Now, strategize ways you can minimize or shift your interactions with these people. Repeat this "energy brush off" exercise as needed.

40a. What delights you? Big or small, silly or profound, which people, colors, sounds, scents, and textures make you smile? Which things can you easily increase in your everyday experience?

40b. Which bigger delightful things can you symbolically invoke (i.e. something small represents something larger, or getting a screensaver/poster/tapestry of your favorite place)? Be creative. Small, symbolic steps create big shifts.

41. Do you feel more motivated by pleasure or pain? Do you enjoy your motivation method? Is it effective? How might these insights change your get well strategy?

42a. Under what conditions do you feel lighthearted, joyful and free? If those feelings were colors, what colors would they be?

42b. What items in your home, closet or other environment echo these colors? How can you interact with these colors more often?

43a. Who or what annoys you and why? Big or small, politically correct or not, be honest.

43b. In a perfect world, what changes would feel like welcome upgrades? What small, achievable step(s) would help you move in the direction of relief?

44a. What's the first thing you experience when you get out of bed each morning? Which sense claims your attention: sight, smell, taste, touch, hearing?

44b. What small shift could you make to foster a pleasurable first experience? Some ideas to get you started: the right weight blanket, fluffy rug under your first step of the day, music, aromatherapy, location or direction of your bed/view, imagining or remembering something lovely. How can you improve your first impression of each day?

45a. Who controls your narrative? You? Your doctor? Your parents? When and how did this story begin?

45b. Reclaim and rewrite any missing parts of your story with you as hero. What do you seek? What noble virtues inspire your quest? How might your journey inspire others?

46a. Choose an experience between ages 1-10 years old in which you felt misunderstood by those around you. Reclaim that narrative. Who are you, really, in your heart of hearts?

46b. How does a more accurate version of this story change the way you feel about yourself? Repeat this exercise for any time period in which others' stories dominate your own narrative.

47a. How do others' potential judgments or misunderstandings affect what you allow yourself to imagine or achieve?

47b. Who benefits by limiting your full expression? Is this a good exchange for you? Why or why not?

48a. Have you ever used your own "failure" as a way to punish someone else? Does your body seem to punish you? If so, for what? In what ways do you allow other people's expectations or projections to affect your own experience?

48b. Who decides who deserves punishment or reward? If it were up to you, what seems fair? If it were up to you, what seems healing? What do these answers tell you about larger patterns in your life?

49a. How much do you value or require a left brain explanation for your recovery? Why do you feel this way? What possibilities does your answer open or close?

49b. If you manifested a spontaneous, full healing - today - would you fear judgment from other people? Why or why not? Would you feel compelled to explain your spontaneous healing, or could you lean into the Mystery?

50a. If "all time is now," how would that information affect your sense of self? What potential might "future memory" hold for the healing process?

50b. As a thought experiment, ask the future (healed) you to share how you got well. Record whatever thoughts, images or phrases come to mind. Explore all answers, even the "crazy" ones. Ask your future (healed) self to recommend books or movies to help you understand.

51. Any trancelike state, whether through meditation, Lyme or insomnia, blurs the line between conscious and subconscious mind. This hypnagogic state is powerful. What would you like your conscious mind to program your subconscious to do for you? How could you experience brain fog as a blessing or advantage?

52a. Which things come easily to you, and which require great effort?

52b. If your abilities and disabilities were guiding you, what might they be nudging you to explore? Try letting your body lead when the mind goes offline.

53a. When did your intuition tell you to do or say something, but you refused? What happened as a result in the short term and the longer term?

53b. When have you followed your intuition even if it did not make rational sense? How did things unfold?

54. Do you believe in miracles? Describe one incredible, positive "coincidence" or miracle that grabbed your attention and won't let go.

55a. How do other people's emotions or health issues affect you? Do you feel them in your own moods or body? Ask yourself, "Is this mine?" Always pay attention to the answer.

55b. Black tourmaline, sea salt, charoite, and hematite crystals all offer protection for empaths. What other tools, crystals, mantras, habits or techniques help you to create an energetic and emotional buffer?

56. How has your family helped or hindered your healing journey? In what ways has their help or hinderance made you stronger?

57. What do you long to create? What wants to flow through you? Do you make time for creative expression? How can you bring more beauty into the world?

58. Where are your genetic and cultural roots? What stories, myths or traditions offer you strength, grounding and courage?

59a. Does nature calm you, scare you, or a combination of both? How does your answer make you feel? What can you do about it?

59b. In what ways could you welcome more frequent positive experiences of nature? Get creative. If you cannot spend time outside, consider indoor plants, nature tapestries or screen savers, herbal tea, stones, nature recordings, organic food and other ways of connecting to the larger world through a small detail. What would help you to feel more in harmony with nature?

60a. If you had a personal motto, what would that be? How has your motto changed over the course of your life?

60b. Do you like your current motto, or would you like to change it? Why or why not?

61. How do you nourish yourself? How has this changed during your healing journey? What parts of you cry out for more nourishment than you currently allow? What good faith gestures will you make towards deeper nourishment?

62. How does sound set the tone of your life? What sounds lift or dampen your spirits? What music soothes your soul? Which spoken words make your soul sing?

63. In what ways have you improved and grown along your journey? How do you celebrate milestones? How do you honor your accomplishments? Expressing gratitude and celebration generate more reasons for gratitude and celebration.

64a. What advice would you give yourself to be a better parent to your inner child? What does s/he need that you haven't given?

64b. What activities, music or colors help you to feel more in touch with your inner child? How can you invite more play and wonder into your life?

65. Who and what in your life encourages your creativity and self-expression? How do you align yourself with creative flow?

66a. Do you believe in reincarnation? Why or why not?

66b. Which situations or lessons keep repeating themselves in this lifetime? Hypothetically speaking, if these were carry-overs from previous lifetimes, would that make it more or less important to integrate the lessons now? Why?

67. Imagine you have access to a time machine. Where and "when" would you go? Who would you see, and why?

68. How could you enhance the time you spend lying down or resting? What would make you more relaxed and comfortable? What would help you pass the time in more enjoyable and nurturing ways?

69. Do you find it easier to give or to receive? Why do you feel that way? What would help you to feel more balanced in this area?

70a. What does your healing journey ask you to release? What does your healing journey ask you to receive?

70b. How open are you to silver linings and blessings in disguise? In retrospect, list five unexpected gifts from a delay, setback or initial disappointment.

71a. Do you find it easy or difficult to trust others? What key life experiences inform your answer?

71b. How do you feel about keeping your word? Do you find it easier or harder to keep your word to yourself or others? How might your answers be impacting your health?

72a. If someone, somehow could gift you perfect health, under what conditions would you accept this gift? Under what circumstances would you refuse this gift?

72b. How might these answers shift your healing strategy?

73. Would you benefit from more or less curiosity, or does it depend on the topic? Where does your mind go? Where would you like it to go?

74a. Have you ever experienced any "time loops," déjà vu, and/or pre-cognition? Describe your sensations, activities and mental state when you've noticed glitches in linear time. If you haven't ever noticed a time glitch, watch some time bending movies like "Sliding Doors," "The Adjustment Bureau," and "About Time." What themes or possibilities recur?

74b. What implications might time plasticity or alternate realities bring to your recovery and life? If you could align with a different version of "you," would you do so? Why or why not?

75. How do you feel about paradox? Do you live in an either/or Universe or a both/and Multiverse? Which perspective offers more opportunities for healing?

76. If you were to create an altar or vision board to represent the healed and successful you, what would you put on it? How big would you make it? Explore different ways of documenting your intentions, and follow up as you feel led.

77a. Choose an object (i.e. a bloodstone crystal or an object that represents your illness). Hold it in your hands. Invite all shame, rage, grief, regret, toxins, and negative feelings to flow through your heart, down your arms, through your hands, and into this object. Feel your heart and body unburden into the object. In a quiet ceremony, bury the object outside or throw it into a moving body of water.

Nature abhors a vaccum, so reverse the process using a rose quartz crystal. Hold the rose quartz in your hands. Feel gentleness, love and forgiveness move from the stone, through your hands, up your arms, into your heart and into all the nooks and crannies you just emptied.

This can take 5 minutes or 5 hours. Go as you feel led. This is for your subconscious body-mind-spirit-soul connection, not the left brain or rational side.

When you want to release metaphysical issues affecting the physical realm, it helps to do something physical to address the metaphysical. The subconscious speaks and heals in ritual and symbols. Keep the rose quartz as a reminder that you have replaced toxins and negativity with gentleness and forgiveness, including self-forgiveness.

77b. When finished with your ceremony, record any insights, visions or affirmations.

This journal ends here, but beyond Lyme, beyond symptoms, your journey continues. I invite you to glance through your questions and answers. How have you changed? What core truths did you discover about yourself? If you feel so led, you can find more information and intuitive coaching support from me at asklaurabruno.com. Whatever your path, I wish you peace, joy and wisdom. Blessings and healing... ~Laura Bruno

Made in the USA
Monee, IL
11 September 2022

13789897R00077